# CARDIAC DIET COOKBOOK FOR PICKY EATERS

## 35+ Tasty Heart-Healthy and Low Sodium Recipes

### Brandon Gilta

**mindplusfood**

# DISCLAIMER

By reading this disclaimer, you are accepting the terms of the disclaimer in full. If you disagree with this disclaimer, please do not read the guide.

All of the content within this guide is provided for informational and educational purposes only, and should not be accepted as independent medical or other professional advice. The author is not a doctor, physician, nurse, mental health provider, or registered nutritionist/dietician. Therefore, using and reading this guide does not establish any form of a physician-patient relationship.

Always consult with a physician or another qualified health provider with any issues or questions you might have regarding any sort of medical condition. Do not ever disregard any qualified professional medical advice or delay seeking that advice because of anything you have read in this guide. The information in this guide is not intended to be any sort of medical advice and should not be used in lieu of any medical advice by a licensed and qualified medical professional.

The information in this guide has been compiled from a variety of known sources. However, the author cannot attest to or guarantee the accuracy of each source and thus should not be held liable for any errors or omissions.

You acknowledge that the publisher of this guide will not be held

# CONTENTS

# INTRODUCTION

D id you know that nearly half of the adult American population have cardiovascular diseases?

Cardiovascular diseases remain to be one of the leading causes of death worldwide. As such, numerous studies have been conducted over the years to develop effective means of lowering the risk for heart issues and improving the health condition of those who already have heart problems.

One of these methods is through the adaptation of the cardiac diet, which is composed of the following elements:
• Fresh and brightly colored vegetables
• Fresh fruits
• Unrefined, whole grains
• Plant-based food products
• Lean cuts of meat
• Healthy fats
• Anti-inflammatory beverages

This cookbook contains a curated collection of heart-healthy recipes that are tasty, yet healthy and fun to make. In addition, a sample 7-day meal plan is included to help accelerate your adoption of the cardiac diet.

# LET'S TALK ABOUT CARDIAC DIET

The cardiac diet is a meal program that is perfect for those with cardiovascular diseases, as a healthy amount of supporting evidence shows its effectiveness in helping prevent those diseases. It is also known as the heart-healthy diet, the Dietary Approach to Stop Hypertension or DASH diet, and the low-sodium diet.

Mainly, the cardiac diet promotes eating healthy and anti-inflammatory foods. According to Medical News Today, a heart-healthy diet also follows these basic principles, mainly what the diet should consist of:
• whole foods
• a wide variety of vegetables and fruits.
• few portions of oily fish weekly
• healthy fats like olive oil and avocados
• nuts, seeds, and legumes

The basic principles of the diet also included what should be limited and avoided:
• processed foods
• (limit) red and processed meat
• (limit) full-fat dairy products
• (limit) alcohol and added sugar intake

For most people, following these basic principles alone may seem overwhelming and challenging. The best approach for this is to slowly and gradually incorporate the changes in your diet. This way, the changes you'll make to your diet will keep you motivated especially in the long run.

Following the basic principles laid out in the previous paragraph, here are a couple of lists you can review to get an idea of some of the foods you can eat and must avoid in your heart-healthy diet.

**Foods to Eat**

Meat
- salmon
- mackerel
- herring
- lake trout
- sardines
- albacore tuna

Fruits and vegetables
- blueberries
- carrots
- spinach
- broccoli
- sweet potato
- red bell peppers
- asparagus
- oranges
- tomatoes
- acorn squash
- cantaloupe
- papaya

Nuts, seeds, etc.
- ground flaxseed
- oatmeal

- black or kidney beans
- almonds
- walnuts
- tofu
- brown rice
- walnuts
- Brazil nuts
- hazelnuts
- pecans
- cashews
- sunflower seeds
- pumpkin seeds
- hemp seeds
- chia seeds
- garbanzo beans
- lentils
- black beans
- kidney beans
- adzuki beans
- fava beans

Drinks and desserts
- soy milk
- dark chocolate
- tea
- red wine

**Foods to Avoid**
As for this list, it's mostly about how these foods were prepared that make them bad for the heart, such as processed and sweetened foods. The quantity of what you eat in this category also matters:

- red meat
- processed meat
- high sugar
- high salt

- trans fats
- saturated fats
- additives and food colorings
- refined carbohydrates

The Memorial Sloan Kettering Cancer Center provided a great food guide categorized by food groups on what types of food are good and bad for this diet. Here's a sample, listing three foods per group for comparison:

| Food Groups | Foods to Eat | Foods to Avoid |
| --- | --- | --- |
| Milk and Dairy Products | Fat-free milk | Whole milk |
| | Low-fat cheese | Cheese |
| | 1-percent | Cream cheese |
| Vegetables | Fresh and frozen vegetables | Fried vegetables |
| | Low-sodium canned vegetables (drained and rinsed) | Vegetables with dairy products |
| Meats and Other Proteins | Lean meat (beef and pork) | Processed meats |
| | Skinless poultry | Organ meats (liver, brains, and sweetbreads) |
| | Egg whites or egg substitute | Whole eggs and egg yolks |
| Fats and Oils | Unsaturated oils | Shortening |
| | Vegetable oil spreads | Partially hydrogenated oils |

| | Avocados | Tropical oils (coconut, palm, and palm kernel) |
|---|---|---|

# SAMPLE MEAL PLAN FOR A HEALTHIER HEART

To get you started, here is a 7-day sample meal plan based on the principles of the cardiac diet.

Note that the recipes for items marked with an asterisk (*) can be found in the latter part of this guide.

Day 1
- Breakfast
    - Wholegrain Cereal with Raisins
    - Soymilk

- Morning Snack
    - Banana Slices
    - Plain Water

- Lunch
    - Tomato and Basil Salad
    - Ginger Pumpkin Soup
    - Non-Fat Yoghurt
    - Lemon Water

- Afternoon Snack

- Dried apricots
- English Tea

- Dinner
    - Oriental-Style Salmon Fillet
    - Apple and Onion Mix*
    - Dry Red Wine

Day 2
- Breakfast
    - Banana Oatmeal Muffin
    - Green Tea

- Morning Snack
    - Fresh Fruit Cup
    - Plain Water

- Lunch
    - Shrimp & Egg Fried Rice*

- Afternoon Snack
    - Wholegrain Crackers
    - Hummus Dip
    - Water with Cucumber Slices

- Dinner
    - Chicken & Green Beans Stir-Fry
    - Greek Salad
    - Dry Red Wine

Day 3
- Breakfast
    - Toasted Bread with Honey
    - Strawberry Slices
    - Plain Water

- Morning Snack
    - Carrot Sticks
    - Green Smoothie

- Lunch
    - Broccoli Mushroom Bisque
    - Napa Cabbage Salad with Oriental Peanut Dressing
    - Plain Water

- Afternoon Snack
    - Banana Chips
    - Plain Water

- Dinner
    - Grilled Eggplant*
    - Turkey Salad
    - Dry Red Wine

Day 4
- Breakfast
    - Honey-Sweetened Granola Bars
    - English Tea

- Morning Snack
    - Dried Mixed Berries
    - Plain Water

- Lunch
    - Pepper Ginger Beef Stir-Fry*
    - Feta Fruit Salad
    - Plain Water

- Afternoon Snack
    - Spinach and Kale Smoothie

- Dinner
    - Mushroom and Kale Casserole
    - Turkey and Black Bean Burgers
    - Dry Red Wine

Day 5
- Breakfast
    - Cherry Oatmeal

- Toasted Whole Wheat Bread
- Plain Water

- Morning Snack
    - Apple Slices
    - Lemon Water

- Lunch
    - Baked Eggplant Slices
    - Lettuce, Arugula, White Beans, And Tomato Salad with Italian Dressing
    - Plain Water

- Afternoon Snack
    - Mixed Berries Smoothie

- Dinner
    - Salmon & Asparagus*
    - Dry Red Wine

Day 6
- Breakfast
    - Chickpea Omelet with Onions and Mushroom
    - English Tea

- Morning Snack
    - Banana Bread*
    - English Tea

- Lunch
    - Taco Salad Wraps
    - Butternut Squash & Turmeric Soup*
    - Plain Water

- Afternoon Snack
    - Strawberry Slices
    - Plain Water

- Dinner
    - Mixed Greens and Orange Salad with Honey-Miso Dressing

- Avocado and Cheese Sandwich
- Dry Red Wine

Day 7
- Breakfast
    - Dark Chocolate Muffin
    - Ginger Tea

- Morning Snack
    - Blueberry Smoothie

- Lunch
    - Cheddar Turkey Deviled Egg *
    - Steamed Asparagus
    - Lemon Water

- Afternoon Snack
    - Melon Slices
    - Plain Water

- Dinner
    - Broccoli and Chickpea Salad
    - Baked Eggplant and Tomato Slices with Parmesan and Parsley
    - Dry Red Wine

# RECIPE LIST

Refer to the recipes below for suggested dishes that best exemplify the principles of the cardiac diet. Each has been carefully incorporated into the meal plan given earlier to give a background on the makings of an ideal heart-friendly meal plan.

If you want to substitute any of the ingredients below, or if you think that there is a better way of cooking these dishes, then feel free to experiment, as long as you will remain within the confines of what is allowable in the cardiac diet. When in doubt, refer back to the cardiac diet food pyramid, and the various tips and suggestions given in the preceding chapters.

## Apple and Onion Mix

Ingredients:
- 1 medium-sized Granny Smith apple, finely diced
- 1/4 cup red onion, finely chopped
- 1/4 cup walnuts, toasted, finely chopped
- 1 tbsp. extra-virgin olive oil or walnut oil
- 1 tsp. lemon juice
- 1 tsp. honey
- 1/2 teaspoon sage, finely chopped
- a pinch of salt

Instructions:
1. Place apple dice, chopped onion, chopped walnuts, chopped sage, oil, honey, and lemon juice in a bowl.
2. Toss until all ingredients are evenly distributed and coated with honey-lemon dressing.
3. Sprinkle with salt to taste.
4. Serve immediately.

## Shrimp and Egg Fried Rice

Ingredients:
- 3/4 cup long-grain jasmine rice washed
- 1/2 cup water
- 1 cup chicken broth, no salt
- 4 oz. large shrimps
- 2 large eggs, beaten
- 2 cups sugar snap peas, trimmed and cut into two
- 1 cup shiitake mushrooms, caps only
- 1 cup carrots, diced into 1/4-inch bits
- 2 tbsp. low-sodium soy sauce
- 1 tbsp. garlic, minced
- 1 tbsp. fresh ginger, minced
- 1/4 tsp. red chili pepper, crushed
- 2 tbsp. vegetable oil
- 1/8 tsp. ground white pepper

Instructions:
1. Combine and boil the chicken broth and water into a small saucepan.
2. Add washed jasmine rice.
3. Reduce the heat to low.
4. Cover the saucepan with its lid.
5. Simmer until the rice has become tender, and the liquid has vaporized.
6. Remove from heat.
7. In a frying pan, heat the vegetable oil for half a minute.
8. Add minced garlic, minced ginger, and crushed red chili peppers.
9. Stir fry using a metal spatula for about 10 seconds, or until the mixture has become fragrant.
10 Add diced carrots and mushroom caps.
11. Stir fry for about 1 minute.
12. Add shrimp slices.
13. Stir fry for another minute.

14. Add sugar snap pear halves.
15. Stir fry for a minute, or until peas have turned bright green.
16. Remove from heat.
17. Add beaten eggs, cooked rice, soy sauce, and pepper.
18. While still off the heat, stir fry for about a minute or two, or until shrimp are cooked through and the eggs have set.
19. Transfer into a bowl and serve while it is still hot.

## Grilled Eggplant

Ingredients:
- 2 small eggplants or 1 large eggplant, around 1-1/4 to 1-1/12 lb. in total, sliced into half-inch-thick rounds
- 2 tbsp. extra-virgin olive oil
- salt

Instructions:
1. Preheat the grill using the medium-high setting.
2. Toss eggplant slices and olive oil in a bowl.
3. Sprinkle with salt to taste.
4. Toss ingredients again.
5. Place eggplant slices onto the grill.
6. Turn over to the other side after about 4 minutes, or until charred spots have appeared on the underside.
7. Continue grilling until eggplant slices have become tender.
8. When storing, place into an airtight container once it has cooled down, and then refrigerate. Grilled eggplant can last for up to 4 days in chilled condition.

## Mixed Vegetable Roast with Lemon Zest

Ingredients:
- 1-1/2 cups broccoli florets
- 1-1/2 cups cauliflower florets
- 3/4 cup red bell pepper, diced
- 3/4 cup zucchini, diced
- 2 thinly sliced cloves of garlic
- 2 tsp. lemon zest
- 1 tbsp. olive oil
- a pinch of salt
- 1 tsp. dried and crushed oregano

Instructions:
1. Preheat the oven to 425°F for 25 minutes.
2. Combine garlic and florets of broccoli and cauliflower in a baking pan.
3. Drizzle oil evenly over the vegetables. Season with salt and oregano.
4. Stir the vegetables to coat them evenly.
5. Place the pan inside the oven and roast for 10 minutes.
6. Add zucchini and bell pepper to the mix. Toss to combine.
7. Continue roasting for 10 to 15 minutes more until the vegetables turn light brown.
8. Drizzle lemon zest over vegetables and toss.
9. Serve and enjoy.

## Pepper Ginger Beef Stir-Fry

Ingredients:
- 6 oz. (175g) lean rump OR fillet steak, thinly cut into strips across the grain
- 2 oz. (55g) mange tout, trimmed
- 4 spring onions, chopped
- 1 small red bell pepper, deseeded and thinly cut into strips
- 1 small green or yellow bell pepper, deseeded and thinly cut into strips
- 1-1/2 tsp. Sichuan pepper, crushed
- 1 fresh red chili, deseeded and finely chopped
- 1 carrot, cut into thin sticks
- 0.8-inch (2-cm) fresh ginger, peeled and thinly cut into strips
- 1 clove garlic, finely chopped
- 1 tbsp. low-sodium soy sauce
- 4 tbsp. water
- 2-3 tsp. sunflower oil
- 1 tsp. cornflour
- 1 tsp. soft dark brown sugar

Instruction:
1. Mix cornflour and water in a small bowl until the texture has become smooth.
2. Stir in soy sauce and sugar until the particles have been completely dissolved. Set aside.
3. In a non-stick wok, heat 1 teaspoon of sunflower oil using the medium setting of the stove.
4. Add the beef strips and crushed pepper.
5. Stir-fry for about 3 to 4 minutes, or until the beef strips have turned brown.
6. Transfer the beef strips to a plate using a slotted spoon. Set aside.
7. Pour the remaining sunflower oil into the work.
8. Heat the oil using the medium setting.
9. Add the garlic, red chili, mange tout, peppers, carrot, spring

onions, and ginger into the wok.

10. Stir-fry for 3 to 5 minutes or until the preferred texture is achieved.

11. Return the stir-fried beef strips from earlier.

12. Pour the cornflour mixture into the can.

13. Stir fry for 1 to 2 minutes, or until beef strips have become hot again.

14. Serve immediately over cooked rice or rice noodles.

Tip: If you are allergic to gluten, feel free to replace the low-sodium soy sauce used in this recipe with any gluten-free alternative.

## Salmon and Asparagus

Ingredients:
- 2 salmon filets
- 14-oz. young potatoes
- 8 asparagus spears, trimmed and halved
- 2 handfuls cherry tomatoes
- 1 handful basil leaves
- 2 tbsp. extra-virgin olive oil
- 1 tbsp. balsamic vinegar

Instructions:
1. Heat oven to 428°F.
2. Arrange potatoes into a baking dish.
3. Drizzle potatoes with extra-virgin olive oil.
4. Roast potatoes until they have turned golden brown.
5. Place asparagus into the baking dish together with the potatoes.
6. Roast in the oven for 15 minutes.
7. Arrange cherry tomatoes and salmon among the vegetables.
8. Drizzle with balsamic vinegar and the remaining olive oil.
9. Roast until the salmon is cooked.
10. Throw in basil leaves before transferring everything to a serving dish.
11. Serve while hot.

## Baked Salmon with Dill and Lemon

Ingredients:
- 1-1/4 lb. salmon—king, sockeye, or coho salmon
- 1/4 tsp. black pepper, to taste
- 3 cloves garlic, minced or 1 tsp. garlic powder
- 1 tbsp. fresh chopped dill
- 2 tbsp. olive oil
- 1 tbsp. lemon juice

Instructions:
1. Preheat the oven to 3500F.
2. Grease a sheet pan with olive oil.
3. Season salmon on both sides with salt and pepper.
4. Combine olive oil, lemon juice, dill, and garlic in a small container.
5. In the baking dish, place the salmon skin-side down.
6. Drizzle the mixture over the fish and spread evenly on top.
7. Bake the salmon until the top is not opaque anymore, about 15-20 minutes.
8. To get a golden brown color on top, broil the fish at 4250F for a minute. Watch over it and check the middle temperature until it reaches 1450F.
9. Upon serving, garnish the salmon with dill and lemon slices.

## Roasted Veggies

Ingredients:
- 1/2 lb. turnips
- 1/2 lb. carrots
- 1/2 lb. parsnips
- 2 shallots, peeled
- 1/4 tsp. ground black pepper
- 1 tbsps. extra-virgin olive oil
- 6 cloves garlic
- 3/4 tsp. kosher salt
- 2 tbsp. fresh rosemary needles

Instructions:
1. First, cut vegetables into bite-sized pieces.
2. Set the oven to 400°F.
3. Mix all the ingredients in a baking dish.
4. Roast the vegetables for 25 minutes until brown and tender.
5. Toss and roast again for 20- 25 minutes.
6. Serve and enjoy while hot.

## Trout Scrambler

Ingredients:
- 1 small potato, cut into 8 wedges
- 1/2 tsp. extra-virgin olive oil
- freshly ground black pepper, to taste
- 1 cup spinach
- 1 egg, scrambled
- 3 oz. trout fillet
- dash of salt

Instructions:
1. Preheat the oven to 375°F.
2. Toss potatoes, 1/8 tsp. olive oil, and black pepper on a sheet tray.
3. Bake until the potatoes are tender, approximately 10 minutes.
4. Remove from the oven, toss in spinach, and set aside.
5. Heat 2 heavy-bottomed skillets over low heat.
6. In a small bowl, combine the egg and black pepper.
7. Put 1/8 tsp. olive oil in one pan, pour in the egg. Cook while stirring constantly until it reaches your desired doneness.
8. Place 1/8 tsp. olive oil in the second pan. Cook the fish until lightly browned for approximately 3 minutes.
9. Flip and cook until the fish are just beginning to flake but the center is still translucent, for about 2 minutes.
10. Serve the spinach and potato mixture with the scrambled egg and fish.
11. Just before eating, season the eggs and fish with a dash of salt.

## Cod Pea Curry

Instructions:
- 1 onion, sliced
- 1 tbsp. extra-virgin olive oil
- 1 tsp. cumin
- 1 tsp. mustard powder
- 1/2 tsp. turmeric
- 1 tbsp. fresh ginger, minced
- 1 tsp. garlic, minced
- a pinch of salt
- freshly ground black pepper
- cayenne pepper, to taste
- 2 cups tomatoes, chopped
- 2 tbsp. cilantro, chopped finely
- 1 medium head cauliflower, broken into small florets, approximately half-inch pieces
- 1-lb. cod, cut into about half an-inch cube,
- 2 cups peas, fresh or frozen
- 4 cups spinach

Instructions:
1. Heat a large heavy-bottomed stock pot over low heat.
2. Add the olive oil and onion and cook until translucent, stirring often about 5 minutes.
3. Add the garlic, ginger, mustard powder, cumin, salt, turmeric, black pepper, and cayenne. Cook for 1 more minute, stirring constantly.
4. Add the tomatoes, cilantro, and 4-1/2 cups of water. Leave to boil.
5. Then, reduce heat to simmer for about 10 minutes.
6. Toss in the cauliflower. Leave to simmer for 2 more minutes.
7. Add in the peas, cod, and spinach. Stir and cover. Leave to simmer for another 4 minutes.
8. Serve and enjoy immediately.

## Mixed Veggie Fried Rice

Ingredients:
- 2 tbsp. of minced garlic
- 2 eggs, beaten
- 1/4 cup of minced carrots and onions
- 1/2 cup of chopped tomatoes
- 1/8 cup of chopped parsley
- a cup of brown rice
- 1/4 tsp. of white ground pepper
- 1/4 tsp. salt
- 1/8 tsp. of ground turmeric for added flavor

Instructions:
1. Cook the rice and eggs separately.
2. Once you have cooked the eggs, slice them into thin strips. Pour olive or canola oil into the skillet.
3. Toss in the cooked brown rice.
4. Add the rest of the ingredients.
5. Sprinkle ground turmeric.
6. Add half a tsp. of balsamic vinegar, if desired.
7. Serve and enjoy.

## Arugula and Mushroom Salad

Ingredients:
- 5 oz. arugula washed
- 1 lb. fresh mushrooms
- 1/4 tsp. shoyu
- 1/2 red onion
- 1 tbsp. olive oil
- 1 tbsp. mirin

For tofu cheese:
- 1/8 cup umeboshi vinegar
- 1/2 firm tofu

Instructions:
1. In a bowl, add the rinsed tofu. Crumble and pour in vinegar.
2. In a separate bowl add shoyu, red onions, salt, olive oil, and mirin. 3. Mix to combine.
4. Add in the arugula and toss to combine with the dressing.
5. Serve and enjoy.

# Cyprian Cheese and Greens Salad with Pesto Dressing

Ingredients:
Salad:
- 2 heads of lettuce
- 1/4 bulb fennel
- 2 cucumbers
- 1 avocado
- 1/4 cup toasted almonds
- 1 packet halloumi/vegan cheese
- 1/4 cup basil leaves
- 1/8 cup dill
- black peppercorns
- 2 tbsp. lemon juice
- olive oil

Pesto sauce:
- 1 cup toasted almonds
- 1 lemon
- 1/2 cup arugula
- 1 cup olive oil

Instructions:
1. To make the pesto sauce, put all the ingredients in a food processor. Blend to smoothen.
2. Season with lemon juice, pepper, and salt to taste.
3. Transfer to a small bowl.
4. For the salad, place the herbs and vegetables in a large salad bowl. Toss well.
5. In a pan, fry the halloumi until the sides become crunchy.
6. Serve salad greens and pesto sauce together, garnished with crunchy halloumi.

## Macrobiotic Bowl Medley

Ingredients:
- 1/2 cup brown rice
- 3 cup chard, roughly chopped
- 1 cup squash, diced
- 1 cup broccoli florets
- 1 cup black beans, thoroughly rinsed and drained
- 1 oz. kombu
- 1/2 cup sauerkraut, chopped

Sauce:
- 2 tbsp. sesame tahini
- 2 tbsp. sodium tamari
- 1 clove garlic
- 1 tbsp. ginger
- 1 lime, juiced

Instructions:
1. Boil 1 cup of water.
2. Add rice and allow it to boil. Cover and reduce heat and simmer for 40 minutes.
3. Remove from heat and allow to sit covered for another 10 minutes, then fluff with a fork.
4. Place beans in a pot with a kombu. Cover with water, and bring to a boil.
5. Reduce heat and simmer for 15-20 minutes. Drain and rinse after.
6. Place a steamer basket in a pot with water and bring to a boil.
7. Add broccoli, cover, and steam for 4-5 minutes then remove, keeping water in the pot.
8. Add squash, cover, and steam for 4-5 minutes then remove, keeping water in the pot.
9. Add chard, cover, and steam for 3-4 minutes, then remove.
10. Mix all the ingredients of the sauce.
11. Serve everything on a plate and enjoy!

## Broccoli-Kale with Avocado Toppings Rice Bowl

Ingredients:
- 1/2 avocado
- 2 cups kale
- 1 cup broccoli florets
- 1/2 cup cooked brown rice
- 1 tsp. plum vinegar
- 2 tsp. tamari
- sea salt, to taste

Instructions:
1. In a small pot, simmer broccoli florets, and kale in about 3 tbsp. of water. Cook for 2 minutes.
2. Add tamari, vinegar, and cooked brown rice. Stir to combine.
3. Transfer pot contents into a medium-sized bowl and top with sliced avocado; sprinkle a dash of sea salt to taste.
4. Serve immediately.

## Stir Fry Broccoli, Onions, and Carrots

Ingredients:
- 1 tsp. light olive oil
- 1-1/2 cups onion
- 2 cups medium-sized carrots
- 6 cups medium-sized broccoli
- 2-1/2-inch broccoli florets
- 1/4 tsp. of sea salt
- 1/2 cup of water

Instructions:
1. In a pan, heat sesame oil to medium-high heat.
2. Sauté onions. Add in carrots, broccoli, florets, and then water.
3. Season with sea salt, and cover the pan to bring to a boil.
4. Lower the heat and bring it to a simmer for 5 minutes.
5. Pour some soy sauce if needed.
6. Optional:
    - Top some pasta or rice with stir-fried vegetables.
    - Substitute other vegetables with cabbage, cauliflower, or yellow squash.
    - For additional flavor, sauté 1 tbsp. minced ginger before adding carrots.

## Banana Bread

Ingredients:
- 1 cup olive oil mayonnaise
- 2 eggs
- 4 medium ripe bananas, mashed
- 2 tsp. vanilla extract
- 2 cups unbleached all-purpose flour
- 1 cup whole wheat flour
- 3/4 cup Brown Xylitol
- 2 tsp. baking soda
- 2 tsp. sea salt
- 2 tsp. cinnamon
- 1 tsp. baking powder
- Optional: flax, nuts, wheat germ, or whey protein

Instructions:
1. Preheat the oven to 350°F.
2. In a large mixing bowl, mix in banana, mayonnaise, eggs, and vanilla extract.
3. Combine the remaining dry ingredients in a different container.
4. Combine both mixtures by adding the dry one to the wet mixture.
5. Stir in the optional ingredients if desired.
6. Place the batter into a couple of loaf pans. Make sure to grease the pans first.
7. Place in the oven for about 45 to 50 minutes.
8. Let stand for 10 minutes. Remove from pan to finish cooling.
9. Serve and enjoy.

## Butternut Squash with Turmeric Soup

Ingredients:
- 1 medium-sized (2-1/2 lbs.) butternut squash, peeled and chopped into 1-inch pieces, reserve the seeds
- 2 medium carrots, cut into 1-inch pieces
- 2-1/4 tsp. turmeric powder
- 1 large onion, roughly chopped
- 2 tbsp. light coconut milk
- 1 tbsp. vegetable soup base OR 1 vegetable bouillon cube
- 2-1/2 tbsp. extra-virgin olive oil
- 2-1/2 tsp. ground black pepper

Instructions:
1. Heat 2 tablespoons of oil in a large Dutch oven (cast-iron pot) using medium heat.
2. Add the onion and cover the pot with its lid.
3. Cook, while stirring occasionally, until onions have become tender.
4. Mix the soup base or bouillon with 6 cups of boiling water.
5. Stir until all powder or cube has been dissolved.
6. Add the carrots, squash, 2 teaspoons of turmeric, and 1/2 teaspoon of ground black pepper into the pot.
7. Cook for 1 minute while stirring occasionally.
8. Pour the soup broth into the pot.
9. Bring to a boil before reducing the heat.
10. Simmer for 18 to 22 minutes, or until vegetables have become very tender.
11. Heat oven to 375°F (191°C).
12. Toss 1/4 cup of the reserved seeds with the remaining oil, 1/4 teaspoon turmeric, and 1/4 teaspoon black pepper.
13. Roast for about 9 to 11 minutes, or until seeds have become crispy and golden brown
14. Puree the soup using an immersion blender.
15. Sprinkle with toasted seeds on top, and swirl in the coconut milk.

16. Serve immediately.

Tip: If you do not have an immersion blender, you may opt for a regular blender instead. Just remember to divide the soup into batches to get the right texture.

## Cheddar Turkey Deviled Egg

Ingredients:
- 6 large organic eggs
- 2 slices nitrate-free turkey bacon
- 1/4 cup low-fat cheddar cheese, shredded OR grated
- 3 tbsp. light mayonnaise
- 1 tsp. white wine vinegar
- 1/2 tsp. chives, chopped
- 1/8 tsp. ground black pepper
- 1/8 tsp. salt

Instructions:
1. Place the eggs in a large pot or saucepan.
2. Pour cold water into the pot or pan until the water is covering the eggs by 1-1/2 inches.
3. Bring the water to a boil over high heat.
4. Once it has boiled, remove it from the stove.
5. Cover and let it stand for 12 to 15 minutes.
6. When it has cooled down, peel off the egg's shells.
7. Fry the bacon slices using medium-high heat in a non-stick skillet until bacon slices have become crispy but not burnt.
8. Transfer fried bacon into paper towels to drain off the excess oil.
9. Once it has cooled down, break down the bacon into small bits. Set aside.
10. Cut the hard-boiled eggs into half, lengthwise.
11. Gently carve out the egg yolks into a medium-sized bowl.
12. Arrange the hollowed-out egg halves in a flat container.
13. Add the rest of the ingredients to the bowl with the yolk.
14. Stir well until the texture has become smooth.
15. Transfer the mixture into a piping bag or resealable bag with a trimmed corner.
16. Pipe the yolk mixture back into the egg halves.
17. Sprinkle each filled egg halves with bacon bits.
18. Serve immediately or after it has been chilled for at least half an hour.

## Go Green Blueberries

Ingredients:
- 2 cups chopped spinach
- 1/4 cup water
- 1/3 cup chopped carrot
- 1/2 cup blueberries
- 1/2 cup chopped cucumber
- 1/4 cup almond milk
- 4 ice cubes

Instructions:
1. Using a blender, mix the water and spinach.
2. Slowly turn up the speed until no solid particles are present.
3. After the mixture has homogenized, add the other ingredients.
4. Continue to increase speed until you reach the maximum speed for 30 seconds.
5. Serve chilled.

## Spinach and Kale Blend

Ingredients:
- 1 cup spinach
- 1 cup chopped kale
- 3/4 cup water
- 1/2 cup chopped cucumber
- 1 green apple
- 1 cup chopped papaya
- 1 tbsp. ground flaxseed

Instructions:
1. Using a blender, mix water, spinach, and kale. Increase speed until all solid particles are gone.
2. Add the rest of the ingredients. Resume blending until reaching the maximum speed.
3. Maintain the maximum speed for 30 seconds before serving.
4. Serve chilled.

## Energy Boost Smoothie

Ingredients:
- 1 large rib celery
- 1 tbsp. parsley
- 3/4 cup water
- 1/2 cup chopped cooked beets
- 1 small orange, segmented
- 3/4 cup chopped carrot

Instructions:
1. Using a blender, mix the water, parsley, and celery. Increase speed until all solid particles are gone.
2. Add the rest of the ingredients. Resume blending until reaching the maximum speed.
3. Maintain the maximum speed for 30 seconds before serving.
4. Serve chilled.

## Green and Berry Smoothie

Ingredients:
- 2 cups spinach
- 2 large kale leaves
- 3/4 cup water
- 1 large frozen banana
- 1/2 cup frozen mango
- 1/2 cup frozen peach
- 1 tbsp. ground flaxseeds
- 1 tbsp. almond butter or peanut butter

Instructions:
1. Using a blender, mix the water, spinach, and kale. Increase speed until all solid particles are gone.
2. Add the rest of the ingredients. Resume blending until reaching the maximum speed.
3. Maintain the maximum speed for 30 seconds before serving.
4. Serve chilled.

## Almond Surf Smoothie

Ingredients:
- 1 large banana
- 1 tbsp. almond butter
- 1 cup almond milk
- 1/8 tsp. vanilla extract
- 1 tbsp. wheat germ
- 1/8 tsp. ground cinnamon
- 3–4 ice cubes

Instructions:
1. Using a blender, place all the ingredients and start blending.
2. Increase speed until you reach the intermediate speed setting.
3. Maintain speed for 30 seconds before serving.
4. Serve chilled.

## Toasted Almond Banana Mix

Ingredients:
- 2 slices whole-wheat bread
- 2 tbsp. almond butter
- 1 small banana
- 1/8 tsp. ground cinnamon

Instructions:
1. Start by toasting each piece of bread.
2. After toasting, add the butter.
3. Add the banana slices and a pinch of cinnamon.
4. Serve immediately.

## Berry Blast English Muffin

Ingredients:
- 1 English muffin, halved
- 1 tbsp. cream cheese
- 4 strawberries
- 1/2 cup blueberries

Instructions:
1. Start by toasting each half of the muffin.
2. After being toasted, add the cream cheese to each half.
3. Add the berries.
4. Serve immediately.

## Berry Blast Oats

Ingredients:
- 1-1/2 cups plain almond milk
- 1 cup oats
- 3/4 cup mix of blueberries and blackberries
- 2 tbsp. toasted pecans

Instructions:
1. With a small frying pan on medium heat, warm up the vanilla and almond milk together.
2. Right before the ingredients boil, add the oats and cook for 5 minutes.
3. Add the berries.
4. Serve hot.

## Apple Cinnamon Smash Oatmeal

Ingredients:
- 1-1/2 cups plain almond milk
- 1 cup oats
- 1 large Granny Smith apple
- 1/4 tsp. ground cinnamon
- 2 tbsp. toasted walnut pieces

Instructions:
1. Heat apple and oats together in a low to medium fire for about 5 minutes.
2. Add cinnamon.
3. Serve hot.

## Energizing Oatmeal

Ingredients:
- 1/4 cup water
- 1/4 cup milk
- 1/2 cup oats
- 4 egg whites
- 1/8 tsp. ground cinnamon
- 1/8 tsp. ground ginger
- 1/4 cup blueberries

Instructions:
1. Start by mixing the milk and water in a pan.
2. Heat the mixture on the stove using medium settings.
3. Just before the mixture boils, add the oats and continue heating for 5 minutes.
4. Mix in the whites, and continue cooking for 4 minutes.
5. Add the ginger and cinnamon.
6. Serve hot.

## Quinoa-Based Oriental Salad

Ingredients:
- 2 cups uncooked quinoa
- 4 cups vegetable broth
- 1 cup edamame
- 1/4 cup chopped green onion
- 1 1/2 tsp. chopped fresh mint
- 1/2 cup chopped carrot
- 1/2 cup chopped red bell pepper
- 1/8 tsp. pepper flakes
- 1/2 tsp. grated orange zest
- 2 tbsp. chopped fresh Thai basil
- juice from half an orange
- 1 tsp. sesame seeds
- 1 tbsp. sesame oil
- 1 tbsp. olive oil
- 1/8 tsp. black pepper

Instructions:
1. Mix the broth and quinoa in a pan.
2. Set the stove to high and place the pan. Let the mixture heat up for 12 to 14 minutes.
3. After heating, cover the pan and wait for 4 minutes.
4. Place the mixture in a separate container and add the rest of the ingredients.
5. Let it cool down before serving.

# Hearty Chicken Salad with Pasta

Ingredients:
- 8 oz. penne pasta
- 1 (6-oz.) chicken breast
- 1 cup seedless red grapes
- 1/4 cup walnut pieces
- 1 tbsp. red wine vinegar
- 1/2 cup chopped celery
- 1/2 cup Greek yogurt
- 1/2 tsp. black pepper
- 1/8 tsp. salt

Instructions:
1. Start by cooking the pasta, a small addition of cooking oil is recommended.
2. Continue cooking the pasta for 7-9 minutes before removing the water.
3. Remove the fat from the chicken and chop it into small pieces.
4. Boil some water and place the chopped chicken into it. Boil for 7 minutes.
5. Remove water from both ingredients.
6. Add both the chicken and pasta together with the rest of the ingredients.
7. Cool down before serving.

## Heart Helping Cobb

Ingredients:
- 4 slices turkey bacon
- 5 cups spinach
- 1 cup sliced cremini mushrooms
- 1/2 cup shredded carrot
- 1/2 cucumber
- 1/2 (15-oz.) can kidney beans
- 1 large avocado
- 1/3 cup crumbled blue cheese

Instructions:
1. Coat your frying pan with oil.
2. Place the bacon and turkey. Cook for 7 minutes.
3. Cut both bacon and turkey into small pieces.
4. Arrange on the plate with the rest of the ingredients.
5. Serve hot.

## Grenade Salad

Ingredients:
- 4 cups arugula
- 1 large avocado
- 1/2 cup sliced fennel
- 1/2 cup sliced Anjou pears
- 1/4 cup pomegranate seeds

Instructions:
1. Mix all the ingredients except for the pomegranate seeds.
2. After mixing well, add the seeds. Mix again.
3. Serve with any type of desired dressing.

## Chicken Breast Delight

Ingredients:
- 1 tsp. dried oregano
- 1/2 tsp. rosemary
- 1/2 tsp. garlic powder
- 1/8 tsp. salt
- finely ground black pepper
- 4 chicken breasts

Instructions:
1. Remove any fat from the breasts.
2. Mix the remaining ingredients in a separate container.
3. Add the mixture to either side of the chicken.
4. Prepare a frying pan, lightly oil the pan, and set the stove to medium.
5. Add the chicken to the frying pan. Cook for 3 to 5 minutes on each face.
6. Cool the chicken for a couple of minutes after cooking.
7. Serve warm.

## Sun Crust Turkey Cuts

Ingredients:
- 2 turkey breasts, cut into 1/4-inch thick slices
- 1-1/2 cups sunflower seeds
- 1/4 tsp. ground cumin
- 2 tbsp. chopped parsley
- 1/4 tsp. paprika
- 1/4 tsp. cayenne pepper
- 1/4 tsp. black pepper
- 1/3 cup whole wheat flour
- 3 egg whites

Instructions:
1. Preheat the oven to around 395 °F.
2. Mix the parsley, paprika, cumin, cayenne, sunflower seeds, and pepper in a processor.
3. Prepare the whites and flour in a separate container each.
4. Coat each breast part with the mixtures separately. Start with the flour mixture, followed by the whites, and then the processed mixture.
5. After coating all the breasts, prepare the pan.
6. Bake the breasts for approximately 12 minutes in the oven.
7. Flip each side and resume baking for another 12 minutes.
8. Serve hot.

# Turkish Meatballs in Marinara

Ingredients:
- 1-lb. ground turkey
- 1/2 small onion
- 2 large cloves garlic,
- 1/4 cup red bell pepper
- 3 tbsp. chopped parsley
- 1/2 tsp. pepper flakes
- 1/8 tsp. ground cumin
- 1/2 tsp. dried pre-mixed Italian herbs
- 1/8 tsp. black pepper
- 1 egg
- 1/4 cup breadcrumbs
- 1/8 tsp. salt
- 4 tbsp. olive oil
- 1 (16-oz.) jar marinara sauce
- 1/2 cup feta cheese

Instructions:
1. Start by warming the oven to 370°F.
2. In a large container, mix most of the ingredients aside from the cheese, oil, and marinara.
3. Mix well and create the meatballs.
4. Sear the meatballs on a frying pan over medium heat.
5. Place the meatballs along with the marinara on an oven pan.
6. Bake for 20–30 minutes.
7. Serve hot.

## Hot, Hot, Hot Salmon

Ingredients:
- 2 tsp. chili powder
- 1 tsp. ground cumin
- 1 tsp. molasses
- 1/8 tsp. salt
- 1/8 tsp. black pepper
- 4 (4-oz.) salmon fillets
- 1/2 orange, juice only
- 2 tbsp. olive oil

Instructions:
1. Mix the pepper, sugar, chili powder, cumin, and salt.
2. Sprinkle the mixture onto the salmon.
3. Prepare a frying pan and set the stove to medium settings.
4. Add the salmon to the frying pan once hot. Cook for approximately 2 minutes.
5. Add the orange juice after 2 minutes on each face of the fillet.
6. Continue cooking for 3 more minutes.
7. Serve hot.

## Taste of Mediterranean

Ingredients:
- 1 cup uncooked couscous
- 1 1/4 cups water
- 1 (16-oz.) can artichoke hearts
- 1/2 cup kalamata olives
- 1 (12-oz.) jar roasted red pepper
- 1/2 cup feta cheese
- 1 cup cherry tomatoes
- 1/2 small onion
- 1/4 tsp. chopped oregano
- 1/4 tsp. chopped fresh mint
- 1/2 tsp. Pepper flakes
- 4 tbsp. extra virgin olive oil
- Lemon Juice from a Single Lemon
- a piece of black pepper

Instructions:
1. Start by boiling water and adding the couscous. Mix well.
2. Turn off the stove after mixing.
3. Cover the mixture and cool for 6 minutes.
4. In a separate container, combine the rest of the ingredients.
5. Place the mixture in the fridge for 17 minutes.
6. Mix the mixture with the couscous.
7. Serve chilled.

# CONCLUSION

T hank you again for getting this cookbook.

If you found this cookbook helpful, please take the time to share your thoughts and post a review.

It would be greatly appreciated!

Thank you and good luck!

# REFERENCES

Cardiac diet: What is it? Foods to eat and avoid, plus planning a diet. (2020, August 6). https://www.medicalnewstoday.com/articles/cardiac-diet.

Heart healthy dash or cardiac diet – what it is | Memorial Sloan Kettering Cancer Center. (n.d.). Retrieved September 2, 2022, from https://www.mskcc.org/experience/patient-support/nutrition-cancer/diet-plans-cancer/cardiac-diet.

Heart healthy diet: 25 foods you should eat. (n.d.). OnHealth. Retrieved September 2, 2022, from https://www.onhealth.com/content/1/heart_healthy_diet_foods.

Made in the USA
Columbia, SC
11 September 2023